This is a book about ideas:

the idea that everything we need has been
provided for us in Nature;

the idea that the body seeks to operate from a
state of optimal functioning;

the idea that we can feed the body nutrients
it needs to be in the optimal state;

and the idea that when we do this, amazing
things can happen.

ALZHEIMER'S HEALING

Safe and Simple by Nature

Karen T. McCormick

3

KL Enterprises LLC
P.O. Box 308, Victor, MT. 59875
http://www.alzheimershealing.com

ISBN-13:   978-1456448615
ISBN-10:   1456448617

Thank you, my wonderful husband, the love of my life,
constant supporter and very best friend.
You make it all worthwhile.

And to my good friend Amy Kraft:
Thanks for inspiring me to do great things.

Contents

Foreword   7

Chapter One: The Alzheimer's Secret   13

Chapter Two: Hope   21

Chapter Three: A Good Night's Rest   26

Chapter Four: Brain Food   28

Chapter Five: The Insulin Connection   33

Chapter Six: Spice It Up!   36

Chapter Seven   Vitamin D3   40

Chapter Eight   The Next Step   43

Chapter Nine   A New Theory   46

Chapter Ten   Update   53

Chapter Eleven   Resources   55

Research   57

Bonus: Help For Caregivers   63

Foreword

This book could have been longer- much longer. It could have been filled with reviews of case studies, research and so on. It could have filled several hundred pages and taken days to read. But for those suffering from the deadly ravages of Alzheimer's disease and related Dementia, time is of the essence. Every day, every hour, thoughts are lost and may never be regained. For that reason, this book gets right to the point.

I'm not a doctor and have never played one on TV. My life has been devoted to being a loving wife, mother, daughter, daughter-in-law, friend and human being who cares about people. I'm a former Army Medic and Psychiatric Technician, Certified Nursing Assistant and Licensed Adult Foster Care Provider who studied anatomy and physiology, psychology and psycho-biology back in her college days.

Health and nutrition have been my focus since age 18- over thirty-five years. The body's ability to heal itself given the right conditions has fascinated me for decades and the addition of supplements and nutritive products has greatly expanded my thinking in this area. This component of the healing process has been my major interest for the past ten years as the ability of simple ingredients we take for granted every day to aid the body becomes better known. After thirty-five years study, it's amazing to me that modern science is just beginning to understand nutrition's true role in the healing process.

The use of proper diet in the healing process has become especially important over the years as time and time again people suffer and die from preventable disease, unaware of the powerful means we each have at our disposal to maintain and improve our health. This valuable information doesn't get to the people who need it because we Americans, as patients, leave our health care up to other people. It's time we start getting educated ourselves on what natural options are out there, because the medical/pharmaceutical industry isn't going to do it. Doctors don't have the time and Big Pharma won't tell you.

For many years physicians have complained that patients don't take their prescriptions, don't follow their recommendations, and don't do as they're told. Until individuals feel the weight of responsibility for their own health, instead of depending on others to tell them what to do, this will not change. The medical industry needs to be one component of our health and wellness system, but each adult must be the one to make personal health decisions, to decide what is best for themselves and their families. Until this happens, attempts to improve wellness in this country will be futile.

Again, I'm not a health care professional. Any and all ideas and suggestions in this material are merely my own, based on the materials I have studied and my experiences pursuing natural health for the past thirty-five plus years. It is highly recommended that the reader follow up, read the materials themselves and draw their own conclusions. It is also recommended that the primary health care provider be involved in this process.

As for the following disclaimers, they are necessary in our day and time. Please take the time to read them. Whatever your health issues, get as much information as you can. It is sincerely hoped the material in this book will be helpful for many and informative to all. We welcome questions or comments, so feel free to contact us.

Conventional medicine can offer little help or hope right now in the fight against this dread disease. It is the families and caregivers who will lead the way in the use of natural solutions for Alzheimer's. To these people, we say, "Thank you".

Sincerely,

Karen McCormick

Note: We make no profit from any of the products or services mentioned in this book. We are not affiliated with any of the companies mentioned in any way. We recommend only because we are confident in the companies and their products.

Medical Disclaimer

All the information provided in "Alzheimer's Healing" is intended for your general knowledge only and is not a substitute for any medical advice or treatment for any specific medical condition whatsoever. We cannot and do not give medical advice.

The information presented in "Alzheimer's Healing" is not intended to take the place of your own physician's, medical practitioner or healthcare provider's advice nor is it intended to diagnose, treat, cure or prevent any specific disease or condition. Discuss this information with your own physician, medical practitioner or healthcare provider to

determine the correct course of action for you to take. Any product that may be recommended anywhere in this material is not a substitute for the care of your own physician, medical practitioner or healthcare provider.

You should seek prompt medical attention for any specific health issues you may have, and consult your physician, medical practitioner or healthcare provider before starting a new nutrition regimen. The information contained in "Alzheimer's Healing" is presented as is and is intended to provide broad consumer knowledge and understanding of various aspects of Alzheimer's and Dementia disease as related to diet and other non-drug alternatives.

The information contained in "Alzheimer's Healing" should not be considered complete and should not be used in place of a visit, call, consultation advice in any or advice of your physician, medical practitioner or healthcare provider. Information obtained in this material is not exhaustive and does not cover every aspect of Alzheimer's disease or dementia and should not be considered a professional source of medical information.

Should you have any health care-related questions or issues, please call or see your physician, medical practitioner or healthcare provider immediately. You should never disregard medical advice or delay in seeking it because of something you may have read here, in print, on the Internet, or any other source of information. The statements in this material have not been evaluated by the Food and

Drug Administration. Any/all products mentioned are not intended to diagnose, treat, cure, or prevent any disease.

Other Legal Disclaimer(s):

Use of Material

All materials included in "Alzheimer's Healing" are protected by copyright, trademark and other laws and are the property of KL Enterprises LLC, a registered legal liability company in the state of Montana, unless otherwise noted. Unauthorized use of such materials may violate copyright, trademark and other laws. Copies that you make of the material must bear any copyright, trademark or other proprietary notices located in the original material, which pertain to the material being copied. Any other sale, modification, reproduction, re-distribution, publication or re-transmission of any information from "Alzheimer's Healing", in whole or in part without the prior written permission of KL Enterprises LLC, is prohibited.

INFORMATION IN "ALZHEIMER'S HEALING" IS PROVIDED "AS IS" WITHOUT WARRANTIES OF ANY KIND EITHER EXPRESSED OR IMPLIED, INCLUDING, BUT NOT LIMITED TO, THE IMPLIED WARRANTIES OF USE, FITNESS FOR A PARTICULAR PURPOSE, NON INFRINGEMENT OR TITLE.

KL ENTERPRISES LLC MAKES NO REPRESENTATION OR WARRANTY AS TO THE ACCURACY, RELIABILITY, TIMELINESS OR COMPLETENESS OF ANY MATERIAL THIS BOOK, ADVERTISING, WEB SITE OR ANY OTHER

Notes

Chapter One
The Alzheimer's Secret

If you are looking for information about Alzheimer's disease or a related Dementia, this is the place. But if it's news on the latest drug trials you seek, you'll have to look elsewhere. If you want to know details of the inevitable downward spiral and how little hope there is, you won't find it here, either. What this book does is ask questions to get you thinking and give you useful information based on science.

How can this be a book about Alzheimer's and not talk about drugs? Or how to cope with watching a loved one descend into darkness? Or how the number of Alzheimer's victims is exploding rapidly because we are living longer and there is really nothing that can be done about it? How can we give information about Alzheimer's disease and not talk about these things? Because this is a book about a secret and about hope.

Hope for healing and for the sharing of this secret with the world: Many Alzheimer's sufferers can get better on the right nutritional regimen. We'll talk about why you won't hear about it in the mainstream news but it's happening anyway. What the various drug-free alternatives are and why they work. This book puts all the details in one place, then adds cutting edge information on protecting yourself and your family from the ravages of Alzheimer's.

Time is of the essence here. Without help, every day an Alzheimer's victim loses a little bit of self, a piece he or she may never get back. A mind is a terrible thing to lose. So let's get started.

A Little History

The first case of Alzheimer's wasn't 'discovered' until 1906. A German doctor, Alois Alzheimer, was doing an autopsy on a 51 year old woman who had died after acting bizarrely for a period of time. He found tangles of abnormal proteins (referred to as 'plaques') in her brain. And so this disease was named after Dr. Alzheimer.

For people in their 50's now, our great-grandparents were older adults then. The incidence of Alzheimer's type symptoms was near zero. Our great-grandparents clearly did not have to worry about this disease. But over the past two generations, something has happened. Now it is estimated that nearly half of Americans age 85 and older have Alzheimer's or some form of related Dementia. The rates for those 65 and older are skyrocketing. Early onset rates are increasing. How could this happen in a short span of just 100 years?

To add fuel to the fire, Alzheimer's disease rates are much lower in rural populations across the world. In emerging nations, despite living longer lives due to increased treatment for infectious diseases, if they have not adopted 'western' diets and farming methods the rates of Alzheimer's in their elderly populations are far smaller than they are in 'developed' countries. If the cause is a genetic mutation, why is this happening so quickly only in countries using 'modern' farming and specific food processing methods? Historically, genetic mutations take many generations to become widespread. So what's really going on?

How is it that Alzheimer's percentage rates in rural, non-westernized areas are significantly lower than in the west? Are WHO (World Health Organization) predictions that the percentages will rise as those populations live longer accurate? What if the estimates are valid only if these countries adopt mass manufacturing and processed foods as part of their regular diet? And what if it is the 'modern' countries that should be looking to simpler ones, more in sync with the natural world, for help with this epidemic?

The Latest Research

As often happens in epidemics, the medical community's ideas of what causes Alzheimer's and what to do about vary. Early research found that Alzheimer's sufferers had elevated levels of aluminum in their brains. Because aluminum and fluoride bind together in nature and we have higher rates of ingestion of these substances through use of fluoridated water, aluminum cookware and antiperspirants, etc. than our fore bearers did, some researchers feel there could be a link.

Others now believe there is a tie between increasing cases of brain disease and our skyrocketing rates of insulin resistance. Some researchers blame inflammation, again caused by our dietary habits and sedate lifestyles. Others think Alzheimer's is caused from a deficiency of neurotransmitters in the brain. And yet others merely attribute it to living longer, a 'normal' side effect of old age, which seems to be the United States government's current take on things.

Big Pharma

Over and over again we hear announcers intone "Because Americans are living longer, Alzheimer's rates are increasing" as if this were a proven fact. Then they launch into a promo for the latest drug "...which can slow the progression" of Alzheimer's and Dementia, showing how much better life is for those that take the drugs, quickly mentioning possible side effects followed by more glowing results and "Ask your doctor...". What really are the side effects of these drugs? Are they worth it?

The commonly used drug, Aricept, lists the most reported side effects in trials as including dizziness, generalized pain and insomnia. (Don't many Alzheimer's patients already wake up at all hours, before the medication?) More severe side effects include hot flashes, bloating, sore throat, and gastrointestinal bleeding, severe nausea or vomiting in 1-2% of people who take this drug. That means 1 or 2 people out of every 100 users will experience this misery.

Other drugs for Alzheimer's have recently been taken off the market altogether, having been deemed 'too dangerous'. Does it seem worth it to inflict this kind of suffering on someone who may not understand or be able to express discomfort?

This type of drug also negatively impacts common anti-depressants, which physicians often push Alzheimer's victims to take because they seem 'depressed'. Wouldn't you be depressed if you knew what your fate is when you have Alzheimer's disease?

This is not meant to be a 'medical bashing' book. But the FDA's policy that only a drug can treat or cure illness, resulting in doctors prescribing drug after drug is frightening at best. Because many pharmaceutical drugs are unnatural substances to the body, they have side effects, some of which can be life threatening.

Consider that a random 2005 study by the Kaiser Family Foundation found 46% of elderly respondents to their survey stated they took five or more drugs per day. Furthermore, the cost of name brand drugs in the U.S. is rising nearly three times the rate of the Consumer Price Index. Spending on Diabetes alone is over 19 billion dollars each year. Clearly pharmaceutical drugs are a money making industry in this country!

And now the push is on to 'control' Alzheimer's disease just as Diabetes is controlled. Not to find a way of curing or preventing Alzheimer's but making it a long term maintenance issue. After all, if a cure is found, a lot less money will be made than if drugs are prescribed to 'treat' (maintain) the disease long term. Part of the push for a maintenance model may also be due to increasing evidence that insulin resistance plays a role in Alzheimer's disease just as it does in Non-insulin Dependent Diabetes. Is this valid?

Diabetes is a real money maker and Alzheimer's can be too. After all, pharmaceutical companies are corporations, and they are responsible to deliver 'value' to their shareholders. Are we being manipulated so that big pharmaceutical corporations can pay dividends to their investors? Hopefully not! But what is causing this explosion of insulin resistant diseases in the first place?

The Role Our Diet May Play

What if you knew that every time you sit down to a plate of pasta with your family, you were inching yourselves closer to a life of Alzheimer's, Diabetes, high blood pressure or heart disease? Are you confused? Doesn't the USDA's Food Pyramid tell us that adults need 6-8 "ounce equivalents" (a fancy way to say "servings") of grain per day to be healthy?

What if you knew that every trip through your favorite drive thru brings you closer to the horrors of insulin resistant diseases? That even a couple of fast food meals per week can cause insulin resistance to be present in the body? That products laden with preservatives and artificial ingredients are even worse for our health than we already know? What if those little children's meals aren't so happy after all?

Or how about that ham? Lunch meats? Sausage? Bacon? Other cured or processed meat products? What if they contribute? What if modern agribusiness is a major player in what causes these diseases, with their food processing and manufacturing policies- how would you feel if you knew that research indicates this may be true and that the FDA and USDA have known there is links for some time yet still promote these substances?

If the link proves to be true, it will cost billions to change the farming and food production policies in this country and the rest of the 'modern' world. Are our governments up to the task? Is agribusiness willing to change? Who knows? For now, our government isn't saying much and putting all the blame on consumers. If the government doesn't take harmful substances out of our food system, are you willing to take action once you know how to protect yourself and your family?

The Other Side of the Coin

All that aside, what if you or a loved one already has Alzheimer's? Is there any hope for the future other than just slowing down the inevitable? Conventional wisdom (and medicine) says, "You can slow the progression, but this disease cannot be stopped". But there's a secret most doctors won't tell you. Many of them don't even know this themselves.

The secret is that people who care about their bodies and look to nature for healing are leading the way in alternatives for Alzheimer's. They are finding natural nutritional options that not only slow the disease without the side effects of synthetic drugs, but also help many people improve and lead longer, more normal lives. Those with Alzheimer's may never be 100% of what they were, but they no longer have to live under a death sentence, either.

This health information is available for those willing to put the time, effort and expense into finding it. What makes this book unique is that it takes all the current nutritional solutions, based on science- real research- and puts them into an easy to follow program so you don't have to do it all yourself. It tells actual accounts of people who have gotten better and continue to improve to this day using these techniques.

Not back to where they were before they got sick necessarily, but enough to do volunteer work. Enough to pick up the phone and have an actual conversation. Enough to go back to doing some of the daily tasks they'd done before. Not a cure perhaps, but definitely better than they were before, better than what prescription drugs have to offer. No side effects, no misery, just improvement.

This program incorporates all the simple food ingredients currently known to improve health for Alzheimer's disease, not just one or two. It gives detailed information on what to take and when. Not expensive pills or exotic supplements, just good nutrition to help the body heal itself. We also tell you why each one works in a way that's easy to understand. It gives you important medical information you must know if someone you loves suffers from Dementia including the secondary disease that afflicts 70-80% of Alzheimer's sufferers and the solution you must ask your physician for.

As stated previously, we are not doctors or other healthcare professionals. Maybe being outside the legal envelope that surrounds the health care profession is what's needed to think 'outside the box' for thirty-five years in the quest for nutritional healing secrets. You shouldn't take our word for it; do your own research and find out for yourself what the truth is. Let this book be your starting point as a guide to making health decisions based on sound research and good nutrition.

Notes

Chapter Two
Hope

This book is created for the average person. It is written in plain, easy to read language. Its purpose is to get out this information to everyone who might benefit from it as quickly as possible. And it's designed so that using the ideas presented here will be easy to implement.

If you are reading this book, you may either have Alzheimer's disease or Dementia, are caring for someone with Alzheimer's, know someone with Alzheimer's or perhaps you are just concerned and are looking for more information. Thank you for including this book in your quest for information. To keep things simple, from here on out, we are just going to refer to Alzheimer's disease and Dementia as A/D.

This book is going to be different from most of the information you will read or hear about A/D. This book is different because most say there is no hope. They say things will never get better. This book is different because it says some people may get better with simple solutions and this book shows you how to do it. It is a book about hope. Hope for individuals, hope for spouses, for caregivers, for families. Hope for you.

We first saw a woman with A/D about 1979. Before then, even though we had worked in mental health and studied psychology and physiology, we'd had only read a reference or two about A/D and had never actually seen anyone with it. It was rare back then.

Ten years after that, as owners of a couple of state licensed adult foster care homes we discovered A/D was quite a bit more common. There were a number of people suffering from those horrible diseases. We say horrible because in the case of A/D, the mind- that which is the soul and essence of the person- seems to die long before the body. It's a sad situation for victims and their loved ones.

Up until recently, there has been no hope and much suffering. The medical community has been doing research and the pharmaceutical community has been developing drugs but no real cause or solution has been widely advanced. While they study and develop, people suffer and die.

This summer, our wonderful, intelligent and highly competent father-in-law joined the ranks of the afflicted. Looking back, the signs of his mental decline were there for as long as three years prior. We just hadn't really noticed it. But over the past year, the fact that something was not right had become glaringly obvious. For the sake of his privacy, we will refer to my father -in-law as "Joe".

Joe had been slipping. He no longer kept track of how his favorite football teams were doing. Despite many years of experience in building and remodeling, he had trouble performing even simple tasks in his workshop. He lost his sense of humor. He was largely expressionless, except when he was angry that people, especially his wife, wanted him to 'do' things.

Friends started asking, "What's wrong with Joe?" They could see that he was not himself. His wife was starting to miss her husband terribly. Their home was falling apart from neglect and botched 'fix it' jobs. He went shopping for materials, but wrote checks for $3.00 then recorded them as $30 in his checkbook- at least he was always in the black financially. And he craved sweets, breads, pastries- his appetite for carbohydrates was incredible.

When it could no longer be ignored or explained away, his family took him to the doctor. His family physician referred him to a neurologist in the city.

The neurologist sent him for many tests. The results of one of these tests will be discussed later in this book. But after a couple of months of testing, the diagnosis came back, "Alzheimer's disease or some kind of Dementia". The neurologist could not be more specific because there were no other obvious symptoms to differentiate his disease from other types of A/D.

All his family knew was that Joe was sinking fast. He had a lot of weight despite his appetite and food cravings. He was losing the ability to carry on a conversation. He couldn't even screw the end of the garden hose onto the faucet. When he wasn't wandering about the house, he sat in his chair with a vacant expression. He even started ignoring his devoted German Shepherd, "Roy". They'd been inseparable for years and the dog doted on his master.

This is where we came into the picture. My husband and I made a commitment that we would be there for his parents; that we would help them take care of their home and property so that they could continue living in the area they'd resided in most of their lives. We were fortunate in that respect- we could do that. Other siblings, many states away, tied to traditional jobs, did not have that option. They were economically tied to their jobs. Each one loved their parents in their own way and each one contributed as best they could. We appreciated the support and assistance when they could give it.

We do live in the same state as my in-laws, though six hours away by car. So we started traveling, one week at home, one week at the in-laws. As my father-in-law faded and we saw the pain his wife of sixty years endured as she lost her husband day by day, we started looking for something, anything that might help even a little.

We have been advocates for healthy living, for healing through nutrition and herbal supplementation for years. The FDA states that only a drug can cure or treat a disease. But we have seen, first hand, amazing coincidences happen when optimal conditions are created in the body. Because we have also seen people harassed, and intimidated by the government for speaking out on these issues, we ask that you be sure to read and follow the disclaimers mentioned previously in this book.

What we found, based on good science and research, is nothing short of amazing. There are nutritional options- safe, functional foods, spices and simple, inexpensive supplements- that may provide some relief from the suffering. No expensive, exotic pills or herbs are needed. Some items can even be found at your grocery store.

Sadly, not everyone is helped, just as not everyone is helped by the administration of pharmaceutical drugs. If one has allergies to any of the foods mentioned, they should not be used. Please keep your physician informed of what you are doing and especially whether or not the foods help (but be prepared for a skeptical response). And remember, we are not healthcare professionals.

We are just people who care enough to give hope to the desperate.

Notes

Chapter Three
A Good Night's Rest

Although this book is primarily about nutrition, there is something that needs to be addressed first. That is the issue of sleep apnea. Joe was fortunate. His neurologist knew that as many as 70-80% of Alzheimer's patients also suffer from sleep apnea. Whether sleep apnea is involved in the formation of the plaques in the brain that are a hallmark of Alzheimer's disease or whether sleep apnea is caused by A/D itself is not known.

Joe's doctor referred him to the sleep clinic at his nearest medical center. He spent one night in the sleep lab, where his breathing during sleep was monitored. It turned out that Joe stopped breathing (had an episode of sleep apnea) as many as twenty-nine times an hour. After seeing the sleep specialist, Joe was scheduled to spend another night in the sleep lab. This time, he was fitted with a CPAP (Continuous Positive Airway Pressure) machine. He would sleep with this machine for the indefinite future.

The machine is whisper quiet with a snug fitting mask. He has difficulty putting on the mask and turning the machine on, so his wife helps him get set up every night. He now sleeps longer and is more rested when he wakes.

Dr. Steven Y Park, MD is one ENT specialist (an ear, nose and throat doctor) who is at the forefront of the A/D and sleep apnea story. He believes that long term oxygen deprivation from sleep apnea could be a cause of A/D. Unfortunately, he also states that he believes using a CPAP machine can stop further damage to the brain but it cannot undo the damage that is   already done. There is a wonderful amount of information on the subject on Dr. Park's web site and it is worth taking the time to read much of the information there.

If you have difficulty reading or do not use a computer, please ask someone to look it up for you: http://doctorstevenpark.com   Specifically, here is the page on his site with articles on the subject of A/D: http://doctorstevenpark.com/index.php?s=alzheimer%27s

Dr. Park practices medicine in New York City, but there are many fine sleep centers at large medical centers around the country. If your personal physician is reluctant to give a referral, either show your doctor this chapter or print out some of the information on Dr. Park's site and give it to him. If he is still unwilling to look at non-drug options you may need to find a more informed doctor.

Notes

Chapter Four
Brain Food

After we discovered Dr. Park's web site, we got to thinking, "Are there other non-drug solutions to Joe's A/D? We knew that the drugs do little and often come with awful side effects. What we discovered next was nothing short of amazing.

Back in 2002, Steve Newport began having trouble functioning. He was eventually diagnosed as having A/D. Despite using pharmaceutical drugs and some experimental concoctions, Steve's condition continued to worsen. He was lucky though. His wife, Dr. Mary Newport, a pediatrician in Florida, noticed that some days he functioned better than others, and started wondering why.

She did her research and discovered there is a theory that people with A/D have neurons (nerve cells in the brain) that are no longer able to derive the ketones that feed the brain through normal channels and the brain starves. It is believed to be caused by a form of insulin resistance and/or inflammation in the brain. There are substances called Medium Chain Trigycerides (MCT) that can bypass this problem. MCT's are found in coconut and palm oil in large quantities. There is also MCT oil, derived from these sources.

Dr. Newport started feeding her husband coconut oil and he began to improve right away. Not giant, "I'm cured!" improvements, but little, day to day changes. She soon began supplementing with MCT oil and the coconut oil. Four tablespoons per day are recommended. Steve Newport's experience, updates and current research are detailed on the web site: http://www.coconutketones.com/

We decided to give it a try. One problem though: Joe doesn't like coconut. And he is not one to take pills or plain oil, for that matter. So we needed another approach. We made a 'cookie' utilizing the oil, (we share the recipe for it at the end of this chapter). Then we replaced his usual soft spread with a simple coconut oil/butter blend. We worked the coconut oil into everyday recipes.

Joe started talking more right away. Two weeks later, he was talking, making jokes, and on the surface quite his old self. However, he still had a lot of confusion. Yet after two weeks on the oil the difference was amazing. He could do simple tasks if someone directed him where he couldn't do them at all two weeks prior. He started to initiate activities. The biggest change of all? He started to care again. Care about others, care about himself. In essence, Joe started getting himself back.

One reason we got such noticeable results so soon may be because Joe didn't get so far gone to begin with. If your loved one has had A/D for a long time, big change will probably take time. Even if all the MCT does is slow down the disease or give modest improvement, it is equal to or better than conventional medicine can offer at this point.

Coconut oil has gotten a bad rap as a 'dangerous' fat. Virgin, unrefined coconut oil is healthy food. In cultures where

29

large amounts of coconut oil are consumed, high levels of healthy cholesterol (HDL) are common and cardiac disease is rare. However, it is our belief that it must be virgin, unrefined oil with its natural constituents to be truly heart healthy.

One good source for coconut oil, Caprylic Acid (derived from coconut oil) and MCT oil is Swanson Vitamins. They have excellent prices and good customer service. They have been very reliable and we are happy with how affordable supplements are through the company. We are not paid anything if you use them. You can also get most of the products at your local health foods store or on the Web. We just like sharing a great deal with others when we find one. http://www.swansonvitamins.com

Suggestions for Use

There are many sources of the coconut fats including coconut milk. Dr. Newport's report lists many good ideas for getting the recommended minimum of 35 grams of VCO into the diet. It is recommended to start slow – a couple teaspoons a day and build up to avoid unpleasant gastrointestinal affects. Some MCT should be consumed at every meal and in the evening in the form of a snack to keep a steady blood level throughout the day. Taking the VCO in capsules is not recommended as it would be difficult to take enough to make a difference. Some researchers believe Caprylic Acid could be the active ingredient in coconut oil which treats A/D. It can be found in capsule form and may be helpful, too.

Using coconut oil in baked goods creates a wonderful, soft product without really leaving a coconut flavor. In homemade pizza crust, it bakes up crisp on the outside, but soft and tender inside. Anything you could want to bake will be delicious with coconut oil. Be sure to read the bonus section for more tips on using coconut oil.

Recipes

Coconut Butter Blend

1 cube butter (½ C) (not margarine or other spread), softened
½ C of unrefined VCO; works best if VCO is soft. Place jar in warm place to soften but not melt. Coconut oil melts at about 78 degrees.

Mix together until well blended and smooth. Measure equally into 7 divided portions, cover and freeze until firm or place in a covered dish and refrigerate. Use as desired anywhere butter or margarine is normally used. Olive oil, which has many health benefits of its own, could probably be used in place of butter.

Keep in mind that any recipe that calls for fat of any kind can use coconut oil in place of other fats. From replacing a tablespoon of oil with a tablespoon of coconut oil to replacing 100% of the butter in a recipe, substituting can be done easily. Because coconut becomes liquid at room temperature, it should not completely replace butter in recipes where a firm product is desired. It may take several tries to get the altered product just right.

Brain Food Cookies

Mix together (food processor works best):
8 dried cherries or cranberries
¼ C walnuts
(Finely chop these two ingredients if making by hand and combine)

Then add:
1/3 C virgin coconut oil (VCO), unrefined
¼ C natural, no sugar added peanut butter or other nut butter
1 t Ceylon cinnamon

Blend together then add:
1/8 C honey

In a bowl, combine:
1 1/3 C regular oats
¼ C dark chocolate chips or chopped chocolate of your choice
¼ C raisins

Add blender mixture and mix well. Place 1/3 cup lightly packed onto a piece of plastic. Fold plastic over and flatten. Or shape into bars. Put into liners in a muffin tin- whatever you desire. Wrap and chill or place in freezer bag and freeze, taking out about 1 hour before consumption to soften. Makes about 7 of the 1/3 C servings, and tastes delicious. Each ingredient was chosen for the health benefits of that food.

Chapter Five
The Insulin Connection

From D.J. Graves at the University of California, Santa Barbara in the following tech brief:
http://techtransfer.universityofcalifornia.edu/NCD/10309.html

"DESCRIPTION: Researchers at the University of California, Santa Barbara have discovered an extract of common cinnamon that contains a class of small organic molecules that inhibit several key processes in Alzheimer's disease. The cinnamon extract inhibits the aggregation of tau and disassembles fibers that have already formed, suggesting that neurofibrillary tangles can possibly be reversed by these compounds. The extract exhibits potent inhibitory activity, is orally available, water-soluble, non-toxic, and the bioactive molecules are likely brain permeable. The extract is readily produced in large quantities and can be encapsulated in powder form for oral administration. These properties make the cinnamon extract a highly favorable substance for development into an effective therapeutic to slow or prevent Alzheimer's disease."

That really caught our eye so we did some research. Slowing down or even stopping the disease with a simple cinnamon extract could be a huge jump forward in treating A/D. Turns out the folks over at UCSB have applied for a patent on their cinnamon extract. Furthermore, they didn't use just any common cinnamon. In this case they used Cinnamomum zeylanicum also known as Cinnamon verum or Ceylon cinnamon, sometimes labeled as Sri Lankan cinnamon. But while you're waiting for the extract to go through the FDA approval process, add a liberal dose of the real thing to the A/D diet right now- and sprinkle some on your own food while you are at it. We'll explain why in a later chapter.

In the U.S., much of what is commonly available are the cassia varieties which have a hotter flavor, but not the tangle busting properties of the Ceylon cinnamon, which is popular in Europe and Mexico. A word of warning: Cinnamon cassia is a natural source of Coumarin, a potent blood thinner, which is another reason to seek out the Ceylon variety. Cinnamon cassia (Chinese, Saigon, Vietnam, Indian varieties, for example) should not be used by persons using Warfarin or other blood thinners. In fact, Germany has banned Cinnamon cassia as being unsafe. However, Ceylon cinnamon (Cinnamon verum or Cinnamon zeylanicum) is considered to be safe for everyone.

Another reason to include Ceylon cinnamon in the A/D diet regimen is research supporting the idea that insulin resistance in the brain causes Alzheimer's, essentially starving the brain. It may be possible to bypass the insulin resistance and feed the brain by supplementing with coconut oil, as discussed in Chapter Three but it may also be possible to decrease insulin resistance in the first place with the right cinnamon.

Studies show as little as ½ teaspoon twice a day can be beneficial for reducing insulin resistance in the body, and 2 teaspoons per day may be helpful for A/D. Because it is water soluble, drinking cinnamon tea is often suggested, but if it's not your thing, just make sure you have fluids with that homemade cinnamon roll.

Suggestions for Use

As a tea or sprinkle into tea as an addition; add cinnamon, sugar and cream to coffee as a treat. Use anywhere you would use cinnamon. Our mother-in-law makes great cinnamon rolls using coconut oil instead of butter in the dough, and uses a liberal amount of cinnamon in the filling. If a liquid caloric supplement is being used because of weight loss, sprinkle some cinnamon in that. Remember to sprinkle cinnamon on hot cereal and coconut buttered toast.

Ceylon cinnamon has a sweet fragrance and a light, delicate flavor, making it much easier to take in larger quantities than the cassia varieties. A little planning should make the incorporation of healthy Ceylon cinnamon into the diet fairly easily. Aim for ½ teaspoon three or four times per day or a couple teaspoons per day altogether. Ceylon cinnamon may also be found in capsule form.

Notes

Chapter Six
Spice It Up!

The next bullet in our nutritional arsenal is turmeric (Curcumin). One of the more curious aspects of Alzheimer's and Dementia is that it rarely occurs among the people of India and the link here seems to be their taste for turmeric. Turmeric has been used in Indian Ayurvedic medicine for centuries. It is anti-inflammatory and a potent antioxidant. It is a powerful tool in detoxifying the body.

There have been over 1,000 studies in both animals and humans on the effects of Curcurmin (turmeric). Turmeric has been used in various types of treatments for dementia and traumatic brain injury and has potential for helping in Alzheimer's disease, too. In fact, research shows turmeric improves cognitive function (thinking ability) in people with A/D.

One reason turmeric may work so well is it's function in assisting macrophages in fighting the presence of foreign proteins and then clearing them from the body. Macrophages are a vital part of our immune systems; they are a part of the immune system's 'clean up crew'. The proteins that are a part of plaques found in the brains of A/D sufferers are in fact, foreign to the brain and body.

One other way turmeric is helpful to the brain is its very powerful anti-inflammatory effect. For people with A/D, there seems to be a great deal of inflammation of the neurons (nerve cells) in the brain. Turmeric protects the brain by preventing and healing this destructive process. Furthermore, research shows Curcumin is one substance that can cross the blood brain barrier and is, in fact, detected in Cerebral Spinal Fluid. Many drugs cannot do this but turmeric can.

Important Information

In the case of turmeric, more is not better. Researchers found the best improvement came for people using small to moderate amounts of Curcumin. In fact, those who ingested large amounts of turmeric did not fare as well long term as the more moderate users.

Right now, some in the medical field believe that in high doses, turmeric may damage the liver and those who are heavy drinkers or have liver disease and related illnesses, should only use turmeric with a doctor's supervision. But Austrian researchers recently found turmeric helped heal the liver in animal studies. This is further backed up by a study at St. Louis University here in the U.S. showing turmeric prevents and/or treats liver damage in certain conditions.

Until more is known, it is best to work with your doctor when using turmeric if liver disease is present. But for everyone else, dosages up to 10 grams (10,000 mg) per day are safe. That's a lot of turmeric, much more than is needed. The amounts given here are safe for just about everyone.

Turmeric works best when taken with foods and particularly, with fats. This is because turmeric is fat soluble. That is, it breaks down in the presence of fats. In India, turmeric has traditionally been cooked in fat with other spices, such as in curry powder, before foods are added. Science has found that Bioperine, derived from black pepper, helps turmeric be more available to the body- up to 2,000% more. So be sure to use black pepper with turmeric as often as possible or supplement.

As the medical community researches turmeric and the pharmaceutical industry seeks to develop and patent a derivative, shouldn't we get the benefits of turmeric that people in India have enjoyed for thousands of years? Adding turmeric to the diet is actually quite simple.

Suggestions for Use

It's easy to prepare turmeric the Indian way while contributing to the daily coconut oil dose: melt some coconut oil over low heat, add the turmeric, and black pepper to the pan with any other spices you want to use. Stir and cook for several minutes over medium low heat before continuing the recipe. There are many delicious and interesting Indian dishes that use turmeric, especially when combined with other spices to make curry powder.

However, because spicy foods or new dishes may not be acceptable to those with A/D, incorporating turmeric into their usual diet may be the most effective route. Suggested uses for turmeric are ½ teaspoon in tomato or corn products, with some fat and black pepper if tolerated. Add a bit of turmeric to potato salad and egg dishes. Adding turmeric and pepper to mayonnaise turns it into a healthier sandwich spread. It can easily be sprinkled into soups, chili, etc.

Add a little turmeric to foods throughout the day for best results. Again, aim for a teaspoon or two total in the diet every day. This is a safe amount that works best for most people. Curcumin is also available via capsule form. Remember though, research indicates that more is not necessarily better in this case.

Notes

Chapter Seven
Vitamin D3

The final nutritional tool we will consider adding to the A/D diet is Vitamin D3. Just like the rest of the U.S. population, many people with A/D have low levels of this vitamin in their bodies. What is unique for the A/D afflicted is that increasing D3 levels may help the brain heal.

Specifically, D3 is involved in assisting macrophages in fighting and destroying the foreign proteins formed as plaques in the brain, just as turmeric (Curcumin) does. In fact, some researchers believe the two may work best when used together, though there is other research showing that some A/D patients respond to the combination, while others respond only to D3. Given the other health benefits of Curcumin, using both may be beneficial to everyone in some way.

The study cited, published in August 2009 in the Journal of Alzheimer's Disease titled, "Vitamin D-Curcumin Combo Offers Brain Health Potential," discusses this at length. The poor absorption of Curcumin alone is cited in the study as an issue. The previous chapter tells you how to improve absorption the natural, easy way.

How much D3 should the A/D person take? The experts refuse to make any suggestions until more studies are done. Meanwhile, real people are suffering and dying every day from A/D. In the US alone, 150 out of every 1000 people over the age 65are affected, with the number believed to be close to 50% of those over 85 years of age.

With these numbers, it seems prudent that 2,000 units of D3 per day could be helpful and certainly not harmful. In fact, this is the amount many physicians take themselves to boost their own immune systems. Up to 5,000 IU per day of D3 is known to be safe. Some people don't absorb this nutrient very well, so being tested for D3 blood level is a good idea. Ask your doctor.

Another reason to add D3 to boost the immune system of the A/D person is for the purpose of boosting the immune system and protect against colds/flu. Because A/D persons are not particularly active, especially in the later stages, they are prone to secondary infections, including pneumonia. Pneumonia is a leading cause of death for this population.

So let's see....D3 can boost the immune system and prevent/remove A/D related plaques in the brain, especially when combined with turmeric and black pepper. Many people, especially those with A/D have low blood levels of D3. Why not start using D3 now? Taking D3 alone may upset the stomach. Taking it with food, preferably with some fat if combining with turmeric and black pepper, is highly recommended. 2,000 I.U. per day should be safe for most people.

If there is any question, be sure to check with your physician and remember to inform your doctor of the supplements being used. If your physician is not up to date on the latest information regarding A/D, you may want to find a doctor that is. After all, the physician is being paid to treat a disease and you and your loved ones deserve to choose from the best options available. With a certain death sentence under the old 'nothing can be done' model, do you really want to follow that path?

Notes

Chapter Eight
The Next Step

The traditional medical route is to do studies, develop and patent drug products, do more testing, and then do clinical trials then apply for government approval for the drugs. Meanwhile, people are suffering and dying, families are heartbroken and the usual prognosis given is a continuous deterioration over time until death. No hope, no future.

Now that we know there are healthy nutritive foods, spices and supplements that can help, should we wait to 'see' what the medical community discovers in a few years or should we take action ourselves now? Should we wait for the family doctor to 'discover' the sleep apnea/ brain damage connection or should we ask-or demand- a referral?

It is our philosophy that when there is nothing to lose, everything to gain and the resources are safe, natural and backed by science, go for it!

We recommend you be proactive and have a plan of action:

1) Ask for a referral to a sleep clinic. You may need a referral from your doctor, especially to be covered under your health insurance plan. If there is a sleep apnea diagnosis, work with the specialists, getting fitted for and outfitted with the CPAP machine. Many insurance plans

will cover most of the costs of equipment and supplies if a diagnosis is made.

2) Aim for about 4 tablespoons of virgin, unrefined coconut oil per day total intake, an equivalent amount of MCT oil or about 6,000 mg of Caprylic Acid supplement. Some actual coconut oil should be included when the supplement is taken since it is not known for certain what the active ingredient(s) for A/D in the coconut oil is. Keep a batch of the coconut oil 'cookies' in the refrigerator and give your A/D person one every day. Start at two tsp per day and work up to four tbsp.

3) Purchase good quality, organic Ceylon cinnamon and work about 2 teaspoons or at least 1000 mg (if using capsules) into the diet every day.

4) Add D3 to the diet, 2,000 to 5,000 IU/day. 2,000 IU will be safe for most people.

5) Use turmeric, aiming for 1-2 teaspoons per day. Take some black pepper with it or use Bioperene as a supplement to increase effectiveness. Remember that more is not better with turmeric.

Please do not read this as an 'anti-medical establishment' work. It is not. It's just that sometimes results can be obtained and suffering alleviated with simple dietary changes. The wheels of traditional medicine move slowly and any drugs derived from these substances will be more expensive than the foods themselves and won't be available for a long time. If we can do something NOW, that will not harm, that may easily help many people (though sorry to say, not everyone), why not give it a try?

We hope you do and that you will keep a regular journal of what the A/D person is taking as far as drugs and nutritional supplementation are concerned and any changes that occur. Keeping track of changes will make sure the small improvements that may be barely noticed at first are not missed.

If you can take video of the A/D person before starting the added nutrition, that would be very good, too. Then take video, on a regular basis, every one to two weeks. The information you document could help researchers.

How long will you need to use this nutritional regimen? Like a diabetic who must take insulin to survive, the A/D person who responds to this nutritional regimen will probably need and want to take it indefinitely. Otherwise, the slide back into darkness may resume. Plan to use the diet as long as you can or until modern medicine finds a cure.

Notes

Chapter Nine
A New Theory

There continues to be billions of dollars spent on A/D diseases. Studies continue to develop new theories on the hows and whys, but little hope for those suffering from these horrible, death dealing afflictions. Some say insulin resistance, some say plaques interfering, some say the plaques are the result of aluminum and fluoride in our diets binding together to cause the plaques, some say not. Another physician/investigator blames sleep apnea as the cause. One recent study even proposes that the plaque formation is actually a result of the brain attempting to protect itself. In other words, nobody really knows what is causing the epidemic of Alzheimer's or what to do about it.

One of the most interesting studies is from a group of researchers led by Suzanne de la Monte, MD, MPH, of Rhode Island Hospital and professor of pathology and lab medicine at The Warren Alpert Medical School at Brown University. This study resulted in a very different explanation of what could be causing the explosion of A/D.

What Dr.de la Monte's research team found is a strong correlation between age adjusted increases in death rate from Alzheimer's, Parkinson's and Diabetes and the progressive increases in human exposure to nitrates, nitrites and nitrosamines through processed, preserved foods and fertilizers used on the crops we consume. Dr.de la Monte and her team believe that Alzheimer's is a disease of insulin resistance and the increased exposure to nitrosamines in our diet plays a significant role in the epidemic of insulin-resistant diseases.

The researchers graphed and analyzed mortality rates, comparing them with increasing age for each disease. They then studied the United States population growth, annual use and consumption of nitrite-containing fertilizers, fast foods, processed meats and fertilizer laden grains. It must be noted that nitrosamines naturally occur in foods and are increased during cooking and commercial processing.

This study looks specifically at commercial additives in our food chain. The findings indicate increases in the use of nitrosamines mirror the increases in insulin-resistance the researchers found. Could it be that our reliance on fertilizers due to top soil depletion and the government's attempt to protect us from food spoilage via nitrates and nitrites in processed meats and fast foods plus our heavy dependence on nitrosamine loaded grains in the standard American diet are destroying our health?

Nitrosamines produce biochemical changes within cells and tissues, and it may be that continuous exposure to low levels of nitrites and nitrosamines in processed foods, contaminated water from run off and our reliance on fertilizers are responsible for the current epidemics of insulin resistant diseases. The authors state that increased rates of Alzheimer's, Parkinson's and Diabetes cannot be blamed on gene mutations. They instead follow the progression of an exposure-related disease.

To quote Dr. de la Monte, "If this hypothesis is correct, potential solutions include eliminating the use of nitrites and nitrates in food processing, preservation and agriculture; taking steps to prevent the formation of nitrosamines and employing safe and effective measures to detoxify food and water before human consumption." Why have the results of this study not been widely released to the general public? Why has our government has been largely silent on this issue?

For one thing, the modern research model begs for this study to be repeated with similar results which takes time and funding. Our government and the medical establishment will not change policy based on a single examination of the link between nitrosamines and health. There have been other studies demonstrating the dangers of nitrosamine use but these substances continue to be ingrained in our food processing system. It is more than just a lack of knowledge which keeps us in the dark.

It has been known for some time that nitrosamines are linked to cancer. In fact, children who eat nitrate and nitrite laden hot dogs three times a week or more have a higher incidence of certain cancers. Yet hot dogs are promoted as healthy fun food for kids. Consumption of nitrate and nitrite laden meats are linked to colon tumors in adults. Ties to other cancers in the body are also suspected, especially throughout the digestive system. Despite knowledge of the dangers virtually all breakfast meats and fast foods in this country are loaded with added nitrosamines.

Why has our government done nothing to get these dangerous additives out of our food supply? Money. Agribusiness is big businesses in most countries as are the fast foods and processed food industries. Anytime food is processed in mass quantities in food factories, especially meats, there is an increased risk of bacterial poisoning. To keep the industry thriving, the FDA chooses to maintain food 'safety' by using additives.

To their credit, levels have generally been lowered to the safest levels possible and Vitamin C is sometimes added to counteract the nitrates and nitrites. But no real effort to remove nitrosamines from our western style diets has been made. Yet other countries use healthy substances where we use unhealthy nitrites. For example, in Eastern Europe, Russian processors commonly use Taxofolin, which is a powerful antioxidant, as a food preservative. Taxofolin may be easy to substitute for harmful nitrates, so why is our government not looking at this?

Finding different ways to get nutrients back into our depleted soils will be expensive and time consuming. Getting the junk out of our water more so. Changing to safe, natural preservatives in our foods will be relatively easy. Because our government refuses to act, we as must take responsibility to do this ourselves, since it's believed to be cumulative exposure over an extended period of time that is killing us.

We are swamped with sources of nitrates, nitrites and other nitrosamines in the world around us. If you are concerned and want to take action, it may be prudent to:

> 1) Eliminate processed meats and fast foods from your diet.

2) Minimize processed foods as much as possible, including processed cheeses and beer.

3) Maintain healthy vitamin C levels, at least 1,000 mg per day, especially if consuming processed foods, as this stops some of the damage.

4) Filter drinking water to remove fertilizer run off and don't use fertilizer on your lawn.

5) Minimize exposure to rubber and latex products, as well as fertilizers, pesticides and nitrite laden cosmetics.

6) Use turmeric in your food and try other beneficial herbs to detoxify the body. There are many quality supplement companies that carry good assortments of reasonably priced products to help protect against nitrosamines and assist with the detoxifying process.

7) Make good use of the Ceylon cinnamon mentioned previously in this book to counteract the effects of insulin resistance in the body and brain.

8) Use turmeric and D3 in combination to help the macrophages do their job more efficiently.

Whether removing nitrosamines from our environment will make a difference in rates of A/D is unknown and is just my opinion based this research. These suggestions are what we do and will continue to do for ourselves and family.

Because of what is already known, taking nitrosamines out of your family's food may be beneficial now and in the long term. For many, this will be extremely difficult, if not nearly impossible. In this respect, we must all look to the future.

That fast, factory made or take-out food you're feeding yourselves today, tonight, tomorrow, next week and so on may create a health disaster years down the road. Is it worth it?

Change is not easy, especially big changes in dietary habits. We already know that even a couple fast food meals per week can cause insulin resistance. We know insulin resistance is very likely involved in many neurological and endocrine disorders. We know insulin resistance causes inflammation, which in turn plays a role in heart disease. We know that long term nitrosamine consumption increases the risk of certain cancers. What else will you have to know to make changes in how your family eats?

To read the full report on this study, see: "Epidemilogical Trends Strongly Suggest Exposures as Etiologic Agents in the Pathogenesis of Sporadic Alzheimer's Disease, Diabetes Mellitus, and Non-Alcoholic Steatohepatitis." Journal of Alzheimer's Disease 17:3 (July 2009) pp 519-529.

Another Idea

What if Dr. de la Monte is on the right track but chasing the wrong chemical? Some research shows that many A/D people have an excess of Glutamate in the brain and when this is blocked, they get better. But where could this excess of Glutamate come from?

A strong possibility could be from the MSG (Monosodium Glutamate) that is also added to our processed foods. This would follow the same, non-genetic pattern of disease as the possible nitrosamine link. Clinical studies in France and Sweden and nearly ten years use of a Glutamate controlling drug in Germany seem to support this theory.

Unlike nitrates and nitrites, which serve to preserve foods, MSG is purely added to make processed foods, which often have the natural flavors stripped out during manufacturing, taste better.

One big problem health minded consumers have is finding all the added MSG in their diets, since there are roughly ten different names this substances can be called, including anything ending in 'glutamate', anything beginning with the word 'autolyzed'. It could be called 'spices' or 'natural flavor' (as in "natural flavor" added to the turkey you purchase at Thanksgiving). Many fast foods and restaurant prepared forms of foods contain some type of MSG. In fact, often when claims of "No MSG" are made, there are forms of MSG used, but the law allows claims to be made to the contrary.

The only way to really know for sure what is in your food is to make it from scratch yourself, using the freshest, most natural ingredients possible. Avoiding the obvious forms of MSG helps, but since manufacturers don't have to disclose what their 'spices' are, there is no other way to insure your food is not contaminated.

Chapter Ten
Update

Time is of the essence here. The sooner you start, the sooner change may happen.

It is possible the reason Joe responded so quickly is we got him started on the nutrition program right after his diagnosis, so he did not have to regain basic skills such as self care, self feeding, etc. If your person has further to go, don't despair. Give it time. They didn't go down hill overnight- the process actually takes years. And it may be months or years before the person they were comes back. Stay with the program. After all, what is there to lose?

Sadly, although many people will respond to one of more of the steps we have discussed in this book, there are some people who do not respond at all. This happens with traditional medical treatments and drugs, too. There are always some who get no relief. It is my belief we just haven't found what their need is yet. There may be many causes of A/D resulting in similar symptoms and we are just now learning about these terrible diseases and what the natural health community can do to help.

Joe still has his good days and his bad days, good weeks and bad weeks. But having good days at all is an improvement; he is much better than he was six months ago, yet it is a constant battle to slow the decline. The genetic component is very strong and his resistance to any form of treatment, including supplements, is a hindrance. The cinnamon and turmeric seem to be the most effective supplements for Joe; we add as much coconut oil as we can to the mix plus the D3 as insurance.

Joe has been talking up a storm and tonight, when my husband gave his parents a call, his father picked up the phone and answered for the first time in months. This was a joyful moment, not just for him, but for the many lives we can help by getting this information out to the world. Please share what you have learned here with the families of those who suffer.

There is still much to be discovered and so much research to do. Many people have yet to hear that there is hope. Our part in this is very small, but if we have helped one person get even the smallest improvement, if we have given just one person hope in the darkness that is Alzheimer's disease and related Dementia, then it was worth it.

We will continue to search for safe, natural nutritional solutions that are supported by science as they become available and we will post updates on research and our journey with Alzheimer's on our web site. Share your story and experiences with nutritional solutions. We'd like to hear from you. Come visit us and check out our blog at: http://www.alzheimershealing.com.

Chapter Eleven
Resources

Help with finding services on the state and local level:

http://www.eldercare.gov/Eldercare.NET/Public/Index.aspx

This is supposed to be the federal government's site to help people find services. On the date we tried it, it was pretty much useless as it showed no results for our state. We don't know if they are working on the site, there is no explanation provided. What we suggest you do (or ask someone who uses the Internet) is a search with this phrase in the search box: "(your state) state senior service division". For instance, we searched "Montana state senior services division" and the state agency came right up.

Or just pick up your phone book and find them the old fashioned way, in the white pages under "State Government" or try calling your state's information hotline and they can steer you to the appropriate agency. Maybe Eldercare.gov will get their program straightened out, but don't wait for it.

The Alzheimer's Association has a very good web site, loaded with information about Alzheimer's. They make it easy to find Alzheimer's and related dementia support in

every state. Unfortunately, their site only promotes using pharmaceutical drugs for Alzheimer's.
http://www.alz.org/index.asp

Web MD is another source of information but like the Alzheimer's Association, although they are informative, they only advertise and promote the use of pharmaceutical drugs.
http://www.webmd.com/alzheimers/guide/alzheimer-disease-support-resources

Dr. Steven Park's web site with information on the link between Alzheimer's and sleep apnea: http://doctorstevenpark.com

This is one of our favorite accurate, drug free health information sites, though sometimes the "government is evil" attitude is too much even for us: http://www.naturalnews.com

Recipes and links to all the coconut oil articles on the Natural News site:
http://www.naturalnews.com/coconut_oil.html

Here's a link to Dr. Mary Newport's highly informative web site: http://www.coconutketones.com

Notes

Research

Cinnamon

J Alzheimers Dis. 2009;17(3):585-97. Cinnamon extract inhibits tau aggregation associated with Alzheimer's disease in vitro. Peterson DW, George RC, Scaramozzino F, LaPointe NE, Anderson RA, Graves DJ, Lew J. Department of Molecular Cellular and Developmental Biology, University of California, Santa Barbara, CA 93106, USA.

Karall J. Jarvill-Taylor, Ph.D., et. al., A Hydroxychalcone Derived from Cinnamon Functions as a Mimetic for Insulin in 3T3-L1 Adipocytes, Journal of the American College of Nutrition, 20(4), 2001

Nitrosamines

"Epidemilogical Trends Strongly Suggest Exposures as Etiologic Agents in the Pathogenesis of Sporadic Alzheimer's Disease, Diabetes Mellitus, and Non-Alcoholic Steatohepatitis." Journal of Alzheimer's Disease 17:3 (July 2009) pp 519-529.

Turmeric

Fratiglioni L, De Ronchi D, Agüero-Torres H. Worldwide prevalence and incidence of dementia. Drugs Aging 1999;15:365-75.

Mishra S, Palanivelu K. The effect of curcumin (turmeric) on Alzheimer's disease: An overview. Ann Indian Acad Neurol [serial online] 2008 [cited 2010 Nov 6];11:13-9. Available from:
http://www.annalsofian.org/text.asp?2008/11/1/13/40220

Bamberger ME, Landreth GE. Inflammation, apoptosis and Alzheimer's disease. Neuroscientist 2002;8:276-83.

Ammon HP, Wahl MA. Pharmacology of curcuma longa. Planta Med 1991;57:1-7

Shishodia S, Sethi G, Aggarwal BB. Getting back to roots. Ann NY Acad Sci 2005;1056:206-17.

Pandav R, Belle SH, DeKosky ST. Apolipoprotein E polymorphism and Alzheimer's disease: The Indo-US cross-national dementia study. Arch Neurol 2000;57:824-30.

Ng TP, Chiam PC, Lee T, Chua HC, Lim L, Kua EH. Curry consumption and cognitive function in the elderly. Am J Epidemiol 2006;164:898-906.

Zhang L, Fiala M, Cashman J, Sayre J, Espinosa A, Mahanian M, et al. Curcuminoids enhance amyloid -beta uptake by macrophages of Alzheimer's disease patients. J Alzheimers Dis 2006;10:1-7.

Ambegaokar SS, Wu L, Alamshahi K, Lau J, Jazayeri L, Chan S, et al. Curcumin inhibits dose-dependently and time-dependently neuroglial proliferation and growth. Neuro Endocrinol Lett 2003;24:469-73.

Giri RK, Rajagopal V, Kalra VK. Curcumin, the active constituent of turmeric, inhibits amyloid peptide-induced cytochemokine gene expression and CCR5-mediated chemotaxis of THP-1 monocytes by modulating early growth response-1 transcription factor. J Neurochem 2004;91:1199-210.

Puglielli L, Tanzi RE, Kovacs DM. Alzheimer's disease: The cholesterol connection. Nat Neurosci 2003;6:345-51.

Park SY, Kim DS. Discovery of natural products from Curcuma longa that protect cells from beta-amyloid insult: A drug discovery effort against Alzheimers disease. J Nat Prod 2002;65:1227-31.

Kim GY, Kim KH, Lee SH, Yoon MS, Lee HJ, Moon DO, Curcumin inhibits immunostimulatory function of dendritic cells: MAPKs and translocation of NF-B as potential targets. J Immunol 2005; 174:8116-24.

Rathore P, Dohare P, Varma S, Ray A, Sharma U, Jaganathanan NR, et al. Curcuma oil: Reduces early accumulation of oxidative product and is anti-apoptogenic in transient focal ischemia in rat brain. Neurochem Res 2007 Oct 23.

Jiang J, Wang W, Sun YJ, Hu M, Li F, Zhu DY. Neuroprotective effect of curcumin on focal cerebral ischemic rats by preventing blood-brain barrier damage. Eur J Pharmacol 2007;30:54-62.

Frautschy SA, Hu W. Phenolic anti inflammatory antioxidant reversal of b induced cognitive deficits and neuropathology. Neurobiol Aging 2001;22:993-1005.

Bala K, Tripathy BC, Sharma D. Neuroprotective and anti-ageing effects of curcumin in aged rat brain regions. Biogerontology 2006;7:81-9.

Chainani N. Safety and anti-inflammatory activity of Curcumin component of turmeric (curcuma longa). J Alter Compl Med 2003;9:161-8.

Kim DS, Park SY, Kim JK. Curcuminoids from Curcuma longa L. (Zingiberaceae) that protect PC12 rat pheochromocytoma and normal human umbilical vein endothelial cells from betaA(1-42) insult. Neurosci Lett 2001;303:57-61.

Mythri RB, Jagatha B, Pradhan N, Andersen J, Bharath MM. Mitochondrial complex I inhibition in Parkinsons disease: How can curcumin protect mitochondria? Antioxid Redox Signal 2007;9:399-408.

Calabrese V, Butterfield DA, Stella AM. Nutritional antioxidants and the heme oxygenase pathway of stress tolerance: Novel targets for neuroprotection in Alzheimer's disease. Ital J Biochem 2003;52:177-81.

Yang F, Lim GP, Begum AN, Ubeda OJ, Simmons MR, Ambegaokar SS, et al. Curcumin inhibits formation of amyloid beta oligomers and fibrils, binds plaques, and reduces amyloid in vivo. J Biol Chem 2005;280:5892-901.

Ono K, Hasegawa K, Naiki H, Yamada MJ. Curcumin has potent anti-amyloidogenic effects for Alzheimer's beta fibrils in vitro. Neurosci Res 2004;75:742-50.

Jorm AF, Jolley D. The incidence of dementia: A meta analysis. Neurology 1998;51:728-33.

Garcia-Alloza M, Borrelli LA, Rozkalne A, Hyman BT, Bacskai BJ. Curcumin labels amyloid pathology in vivo, disrupts existing plaques and partially restores distorted neurites in an Alzheimer mouse model. J Neurochem 2007;102:1095-104.

Fiala M, Liu PT, Espinosa-Jeffrey A, Rosenthal MJ, Bernard G, Ringman JM, et al. Innate immunity and transcription of MGAT-III and Toll-like receptors in Alzheimers disease patients are improved by bisdemethoxycurcumin. Proc Natl Acad Sci USA 2007;104:12849-54.

Shoba G, Joy D, Joseph T, Majeed M, Rajendran R, Srinivas PS. Influence of piperine on the pharmacokinetics of curcumin in animals and human volunteers. Planta Med 1998;64:353-6.

Rasyid A, Rahman AR, Jaalam K, Lelo A. Effect of different curcumin dosages on human gall bladder. Asia Pac J Clin Nutr 2002;11:314-8.

Lim GP, Chu T, Yang F, Beech W, Frautschy SA, Cole GM The curry spice curcumin reduces oxidative damage and amyloid pathogenesis on Alzheimer's transgenic mouse. J Neurosci 2001;21:8370-7.

Wu A, Ying Z, Gomez-Pinilla F. Dietary curcumin counteracts the outcome of traumatic brain injury on oxidative stress, synaptic plasticity and cognition. Exp Neurol 2006;197:309-17.

Ringman JM, Frautschy SA, Cole GM, Masterman DL, Cummings JL. A potential role of the curry spice curcumin in Alzheimer's disease. Curr Alzheimer Res 2005;2:131-6.

Cheng A, Saint Louis University (2010, October 30). Spice in curry could prevent liver damage. Findings published in the September, 2010 issue of *Endocrinology*.

Notes

Bonus Section
Help For Caregivers

This is by no means the definitive guide for caregivers, merely suggestions for dealing with common problems that have worked for me in the past. Hopefully it can be helpful to others. In any event, your medical team should be your first line of defense in caring for the A/D person.

TOPICS

DIET
MOOD
BEHAVIOR
EXERCISE
HEALTH
TRAVEL
CAREGIVING
LEGAL ISSUES
CONCLUSION

DIET

Anytime the body is trying to rid itself of disease or abnormality, optimal nutrition is needed. The healing process cannot take place without the proper fuel. One of the big issues for A/D caregivers is dealing with food cravings and changing eating habits. Another is excessive weight loss or weight gain. Let's talk about these concerns.

It has long been known that women have food cravings during pregnancy and science has linked many of those cravings to nutritional deficiencies. Could it be that food cravings in A/D persons are also linked to deficiencies? It is not known, but it was our observation that Joe craved carbohydrates in the early stages of the disease. Anything sweet and full of grains, such as wheat or oats was fair game. He often ate six pieces of toast for breakfast along with a bowl of oatmeal topped with honey and raisins. Copious amounts of jam and margarine were spread on the toast. Snacks were often sweet rolls or candy bars.

Despite his high caloric intake, Joe's body was shrinking just as his brain was shrinking (as shown on his brain scan). It was as if he couldn't get enough fuel into his system. When the link between insulin resistance in the brain and A/D came to our attention, it all made sense. We tried the coconut oil route as an alternate path to feed the brain and rapidly began to see improvements. Joe improved because his brain was literally starving and that need was met. We then started adding the Ceylon cinnamon in hopes of counteracting some of the insulin resistance in both the brain and the body.

Joe had lost a lot of weight that his fit and trim body to not have the leeway to lose. Once his carbohydrate cravings diminished and mood, emotions and level of comprehension improved, we could address the weight loss more easily. Before that time, Joe was resistant to making any changes in his diet. Joe was now often satisfied with his usual two pieces of toast with eggs or oatmeal for breakfast.

We added a nutritional drink combined with scoops of ice cream as 'shake' every day, adding an extra 500 calories per day. The goal is to increase calories without adding a lot of unhealthy fat to the body, so we will work on increases slowly. Our next effort will be to add more protein to Joe's diet, to aid in the rebuilding of lost muscle as Joe becomes more healthy and active again. We will focus on boosting the high antioxidant fruits and vegetables to his diet. Since A/D people have difficulty with change, we will work on improving his diet based on what his dietary preferences have been most of his adult life, but in a healthier way.

Let us reiterate that we not medical professionals or licensed nutritionists by any account. We are just people who care deeply about alleviating human suffering and guiding people through the nutritional maze. Many people are interested in finding ways to heal through natural foods and supplements, with little or no harmful side effects. The information is out there for those who have time, energy and resources to search. For those who don't, we've written this book.

If your A/D person has food cravings, it may be helpful to look at what they are and consider what nutrients in the body he/she may be lacking. A consult with a naturopathic physician may be very helpful. Doing this is part of being a participant in the health care process, not just a passive recipient of 'orders'. You have a role to play as a caregiver and a big part of that is to do everything you can to fight this disease for your loved one.

Not that you should go against doctor's orders, but fill in the gaps that health care professionals may miss and be part of the group pursuing non-drug solutions for this deadly disease. History has shown that the natural health community has to fight to get acceptance for using natural solutions, until the standard medical community takes notice. Chances are that if you decide to use natural, safe and healthy alternatives for A/D, you will experience opposition from traditional medical practitioners, who still believe nothing can be done for A/D.

Because sometimes having a ravenous appetite and little self control leads to big weight gains, looking at calorie reduction may be necessary. If you are too obvious about it, the recipient of the 'diet' may object- it's a change, after all. Calorie reduction can be a simple as using smaller dishes and/or slightly smaller portions. Removing excessive sugars and fats from recipes can also help; as much as 25% can be cut with little discernible difference. Substituting a lower calorie/fat ingredient for a high calorie/fat one may be helpful, too.

Another way to decrease/increase calories is to make it a group effort, especially if there is a great deal of suspicion from the A/D person. "We're all working on getting healthier, so we are cutting some of the junk" will probably get you a lot farther than "You've gained so much weight, you've got to go on a diet."

One issue we've run across implementing the nutritional program is being consistent with the program, especially if using the spices as additions to food versus taking them in supplement form. Cooks who have followed recipes carefully for years may balk at making changes or not think about adding extra spices to the dish at all. Taking a supplement form with meals would probably be the most effective way to get the correct doses of Cinnamon verum or turmeric into the diet, but not everyone is comfortable taking

66

pills. And these spices can help make food more palatable if the sense of taste is still present.

Getting the coconut oil into foods can sometimes be another issue. Dr. Newport recommends four tablespoons of coconut oil or MCT oil per day. It can be mixed in equal parts with butter (using margarine or other fake 'spreads' is NOT advised) for table use or used straight in recipes with little discernible difference. It can be used in place of or with olive oil. Any place a fat is needed, coconut oil can do the job.

Because coconut oil liquefies at about 78 degrees, just sitting in a sunny window may make the solid oil easy to work with. Conversely, adding cold ingredients on top of the oil before mixing can make it suddenly turn hard and difficult to incorporate. Mixing the coconut oil into dry ingredients before adding other liquids on top of it and making sure the mix itself is at least room temperature helps. A food processor makes this job easy.

Dr. Newport recommends adding either a (high quality) fish oil supplement or oily fish to the diet to have a good balance of the proper healthy fats. While fresh salmon is very expensive in many areas and farmed salmon can be high in carcinogenic PCB's, canned wild salmon is an affordable, convenient and easy to use choice. Serving salmon, sardines, or other oily fish once or twice a week in lieu of a supplement can be a good idea.

And remember: All things in moderation, as nutritional foods, in their purest, most natural form possible.

MOOD

Having a blank, expressionless face is also common in A/D and is referred to as having a "flat affect" in the psychiatric community. As the A/D person loses more of him or her self, this becomes more common.

Common moods in the earlier stages of A/D are anger and hostility, an unwillingness to accept help. People who have been competent to take care of themselves their entire adult lives now find other people wanting to step in and take over. They don't understand why people want to do that. They get irritated that people just won't let them do things themselves even though what they are doing may make no sense to others.

They often resist any changes in their world. This may be because learning new things is difficult, if not impossible, if one has A/D. Many people can remember clearly what they did forty years ago, but can't remember what they had for lunch just a couple hours ago. This must be considered whenever looking to make a change. Big sudden changes will probably be met with resistance; small gradual changes will be easier for everyone involved.

For instance, if a move is required, exposing the A/D person to the new location prior to the move in the form of short visits, gradually lengthening until the final complete move will make the transition easier. If the move will involve new caregivers, the current caregiver should remain throughout the first few visits, with the new caregiver gradually taking over.

Of course, this all works only if big changes can be done slowly. If not, try to keep things as familiar as possible, introduce changes in small increments and expect some agitation and confusion to occur. The more the situation can be kept familiar, the better it will be.

Depression is another mood that is common in A/D, especially in the early stages when the A/D person is aware that something is happening, but doesn't know what, and/or just after diagnosis when the person may be very upset and feel hopeless.

There is some research-based evidence that a deficiency in vitamin D3 can be related to depression. It is known that A/D persons tend to be deficient in this vitamin. Because they also tend to have decreased immune function and D3 is known to improve immune function and mood, supplementing with a healthy dose of D3 is probably an excellent idea that is safe at 2,000 IU per day or as your physician recommends.

Exercise, getting outdoors and exposure to sunlight or natural light simulating lamps are also natural drug free depression relievers. Other herbal products for depression are not recommended in this instance as they may interact with prescription drugs and alcohol.
For many people, however, just having someone who cares, someone to reassure them that they won't go through A/D alone is what is needed most.

Imagine what it must be like to have A/D. It's like waking up in a city in some foreign country, where most people don't speak your language, the printed word is difficult to decipher and the world is a strange and confusing place. Every week you venture further and further away from the city, further away from people you know, language you understand, and your world keeps getting stranger and stranger. The habits you've practiced your entire life no longer work and your world no longer makes sense. And you are doing this alone. You may have a guide, but there is no one familiar taking this journey with you. That is what A/D is like for those living it.

One important thing to remember is that A/D people are very affected by the moods, stress levels and behaviors of the people around them. If you are stressed, they will be, too. If your spouse is angry that your A/D person is taking up so much of your time, they will pick up on that anger. It's very difficult at times to keep things relaxed and low key, but doing so, especially when conditions are creating stress, can prevent some of the moods that create behavior issues.

BEHAVIOR

It's the strange behavior of A/D persons that often brings their disease to the attention of family and friends. For instance, one woman's mother put a lamp behind the dryer, because in her mind, lamps put out heat and the dryer needed heat to dry the clothes- it's these strange and convoluted associations that feed the sometimes bizarre behaviors in the world of A/D. We realized there was something seriously wrong with Joe when he fixed a burned out headlamp in his truck by completely disassembling all the headlights, then carefully taping them back in place with duct tape, totally covering the lenses.

Sometimes the people who associate with the person on a regular basis get so accustomed to their strange behavior that it becomes their norm and it's not until a casual acquaintance asks, "What's wrong with Ralph?" that they even start to notice that something IS wrong, very WRONG.

Simple tasks and learned skills fall away. Behavior becomes more bizarre, more different and many of the social graces are left behind. It does no good to remind the A/D afflicted to be polite; they don't know what 'polite' is anymore. Because of this and poor tolerance of all things new, social activities are often best limited to family and close friends.

Distrust and paranoia are common, especially in the middle stages. For the A/D person, their world seems to be spinning out of control. The person believes that people are talking and plotting behind his or her back. Some of it may be imagined. But it is often true to a certain extent, because the nature of the disease itself requires conversation amongst family members, caregivers and medical personnel. People have to talk about how to best take care of the A/D person, and he/she may not enjoy being the topic of conversation. When discussing matters regarding the A/D person, it is usually better to do so privately.

You might think it would be better to discuss things with the A/D person present and involved. Just one problem- they often won't admit anything is wrong when they are feeling confused, don't see the need to do anything different, don't want to do anything, period and get angry at being the topic of discussion! Any discussion with the A/D individual present should be very low key and be prepared to drop the subject until a time when conversation comes easier. Forcing the issue seldom helps.

Dealing with angry behavior is real issue here. He/she may lash out at loved ones, especially when frustrated or confused. Anger may develop over being "told what to do" despite the clear need for direction and assistance. One important piece of advice is to remember it is the disease, not the person causing this and often stepping away, even if it means leaving things undone, will diffuse the situation. Of course, this should not happen where safety is concerned. But letting the person decide what he/she wants to do when it comes to non-essential issues can bring about a change in mood. Keeping a calm and relaxed attitude yourself really does help, too.

Another cause of anger or irritability is being asked questions. Questions are difficult for the A/D person to answer. Being asked questions is very stressful when you can't come up with an answer. A question that has a simple "yes" or "no' answer can be best question to ask. Some people would rather be asked no questions at all.

Sometimes just a simple calming action such as turning down the volume of the television or changing channels to a more relaxing program can help. Decreasing clutter in a room and simplifying the surroundings can be beneficial, too. One of the most relaxing colors is purported to be pale pink. While we may be skeptical of such things, making just a small change in a room can be calming.

Some people develop the habit of undressing in public. Often it can be prevented by dressing in sweat pants, fastened snugly with a pull over top. But then again, I have heard of caregivers resorting to jumpsuits put on backwards, so as to make undressing one's self virtually impossible. The key here, as with many things related to being an A/D caregiver, is to find creative solutions that work for you.

Wandering is a real safety issue in later stages. Fortunately, most hardware stores now sell easy to install door alarms.

Adding an additional lock, such as a simple hinge lock in an unexpected place on the door may also be useful to stop the wander from going outside unattended. However, if the A/D person wandering keeps the caregiver from getting sufficient rest, it may be time to consider getting outside help. Your state senior services division should be able to give you guidance on this.

Novel approaches to the issue of wandering include placing a black rug in front of exits- it seems A/D people interpret this as a hole to be avoided. Others have staff greet would be escapees near exits to distract them. Some care homes have placed' bus stops' near exits in case residents do wander out as they may stop and wait there instead of walking off. While installing a fake bus stop is probably not an option, a black rug in front of an exit may be a low cost, low stress deterrent.

ID bracelets and high tech GPS enabled tracking devices are really important if keeping the person in the house is an issue. Your doctor or pharmacist can steer you to resources or visit Brickhouse Security, a retailer with a variety of safety products for sale on the Web.
www.brickhousesecurity.com

Be proactive on this; don't wait until a wanderer has gotten lost to take action. Every year we hear tragic stories of confused people who have gotten lost; often their bodies are found months later by accident.

Persons with A/D should never cook or use any tools unsupervised. Keeping an A/D person safe can be a full time job. Not only do we have to protect them from themselves, we have to protect innocent people who wander into their paths, too. Power tools, hot burners, scalding faucets, firearms and more. Anything that could seriously injure them or you must be removed from the A/D person's reach when they can no longer use them safely. It is better to err on the side of caution in this matter than to regret not having done something sooner.

A huge issue is driving. Driving represents being competent and independent. Being dependent on someone else to provide transportation is difficult for older adults who are proud of their vehicles and driving ability. When to stop driving is difficult to know. But consider that driving impaired is driving impaired whether it's under the influence of alcohol or under the influence of A/D. A person who cannot operate simple tools safely should not be operating something that could kill innocent bystanders. In fact, recent studies suggest that drivers over the age of 85 with impaired thinking have four times the accident rate of teens.

Families often balk at being the ones to take away the keys. Physicians can do families a real favor if they 'order' the person to quit driving. It's not easy to enforce a 'no driving' rule when the recipient is angry and one has to live with them everyday. Having an authority figure make the decision takes some of that burden off caregivers. Many doctors don't like having to be the 'bad guy', but if families request help physicians should be willing to do so.

Another way to deal with the driving issue is to have the person's driving ability evaluated by a specialist, usually an Occupational Therapist. A variety of tests will be given, including a driving test. If the individual is unwilling to accept the results of the testing, contact your state driver's licensing agency.

We have only touched on a few of the behavioral issues A/D caregivers face. Always be safe above all else. Joining your local A/D caregiver's group can be a real help. It's good to have support and helpful tips from others who are going through the same thing you are. Please be aware, however, that if you mention using nutrition to help, they may think you are a bit strange and even try to discourage you. But science is on your side. If you want to use nutritional healing with safe foods and spices, it is perfectly alright to add them to the diet. But please, always keep your physician in the loop.

EXERCISE

Maintaining physical activity is important for A/D people. Being sedate causes muscles to atrophy. A/D people are more prone to pneumonia, partly due to inactivity. And staying active improves stamina and stability. But what kind of exercise is appropriate for those with Alzheimer's? That really depends on what the person can handle. The activity should be tailored to the person's condition and habits. A lifelong tennis player or golfer may enjoy getting out and 'hitting a few'. Fishing may not be much exercise, but for a devoted fisherman, going out to the lake and casting a line may be helpful in keeping him active and engaged in life.

If the person is able to walk safely, exercising the legs in a familiar neighborhood, or even time spent walking in the back yard is good, especially if it's a sunny day (But don't over do it- check that the person's medications will not make them prone to burning easily before you get them out into the sun.) They should be accompanied on those walks. Be sure supervision is adequate for the person's needs.

For someone who is not so confused as to wander, then spending time alone in the back yard can be soothing break from the constant stress of our noisy world. Even an A/D person needs some time to unwind. Just discreetly watching out a window may be all the supervision that's needed. If you are not sure, err on the side of caution. Don't send a wanderer out to the back yard to get some fresh air alone.

Some people have difficulty maintaining good balance. For these, simple stretches or even lifting small weights while sitting in a chair will be helpful. Many local PBS (Public Broadcasting System) have weekday or weekend morning exercise programs geared toward the elderly/disabled. For DVD, try Mary Ann Wilson's award winning "Sit and be Fit" program available on her web site: http://www.sitandbefit.org There is information specific to Alzheimer's and exercise, as well as other health challenges seniors may experience. Above all else, you just need to keep your A/D person physically active in whatever way he or she can.

HEALTH

You must work as a team with your health care providers. The caregiver(s) see the A/D person more than anyone else. Your input will be crucial when that person cannot speak for him or her self. You must learn to notice the small things, because it is the small things that precede the big things.

For example, a normally active person may become very inactive and quiet when illness comes on or may become abnormally agitated for no apparent reason. Any change from the usual behavior is cause for concern. Other signs may be physical symptoms. Because A/D people may be immune compromised, every sign of illness should be

76

reported to the physician as soon as it is noticed and if the person is clearly in distress, do not hesitate to seek health care immediately.

Getting flu and pneumonia vaccinations are a good idea, but if the person is resistant to getting a shot, then those who are normally around him/her should get them and any one who is ill should not visit as even a simple cold can be disastrous for the A/D person. Remember good hand washing for everyone involved, too. Don't just practice it, insist on it. Stop bacteria and viruses before they get a chance to spread disease.

Maintaining good hygiene is often difficult as the disease progresses. Sometimes having a trained nursing assistant come in a couple times a week as the 'bath person' can help, as opposed to fighting family members over having to clean up.

Dental care is still important. If a dentist is needed, look for someone with experience caring for A/D people. When using a toothbrush is no longer an option, using prepackaged dental sponges or even wiping the teeth with a moist cloth can help clean the teeth and freshen breath. Remember to clean the tongue, too.

When nutrition is an issue, consider adding vitamin packed nutritional drinks to the diet. Be careful not to confuse nutritional support drinks with the weight loss ones! Common brands of nutritional support include "Boost" and "Ensure". Ensure is available in a higher calorie version if adding calories is needed. Many 'Big Box' chain stores have their own version of Ensure, which are just as nutritionally complete as the name brand. These drinks are usually sold in the pharmacy area of stores.

Constipation can be an issue, too, especially with poor eating habits and lack of exercise. Be sure to tell your doctor if this is an issue. A stool softener can be prescribed as well as a source of added fiber. The newer clear fiber products that can be added to regular foods can be very helpful as are the old standbys of prune juice and bran cereals. Be sure plenty of fluids are being consumed. Dehydration is a cause of constipation and other health issues.

Another important health issue for many A/D people is difficulty swallowing pills, especially in the later stages of the disease. Surprisingly, giving medications with applesauce instead of fluids works very well.

If choking on liquids becomes a concern, ask your doctor for a referral to a swallowing therapist, such as a speech pathologist. Using thickeners for liquids is often the recommended course of action. These products can be added to liquids, which can then be eaten with a spoon. Thickeners are usually derived from corn starch. One brand of this product is "Thicken Up" by Nestle. Hormel Health Labs also has a line of thickeners and both companies offer ready to use beverages. They can be ordered on line and may be found at medical supply stores, too.
Sources:

http://www.nestlenutritionstore.com

http://www.hormelhealthlabs.com

TRAVEL

Sometimes, as the disease progresses, the A/D person will decide he must take a trip to see an old acquaintance or visit some long forgotten place. This is not the same as taking in favorite spots or reliving old memories one last time early in the disease. Those sorts of trips are good if one can do it without breaking the bank. Compulsive trips are not.

In later stages, it is often the case that the reason for going is forgotten once the destination is reached. After considerable planning, time, expense and trouble, many caregivers find it would have been better to have just stayed home. Don't fall for the insistent demand. It is often the idea of the moment. Redirecting to other tasks or just taking a short trip around your neighborhood or town may be enough to satisfy for the moment. And the resourceful person can usually find a reason not to go that will be accepted.

As a rule, A/D persons do not travel well because travel is new; it's unpredictable for them and very stressful. If the person has always traveled by car, now is not the time to take up air travel. In fact, with the new security measures involving pat downs which the A/D person may not understand, air travel may not be a good idea at all. Try to keep all travel short, relaxed and as easy as possible.

Caregivers often find it is easier when they must travel to hire a respite care person than it is to take the A/D person on long trips. Although the A/D person may be unhappy to be left behind especially at first, if the respite care person is liked it soon gets to be a treat. In fact, cooking the person's favorite foods or doing fun activities are good ways for the respite care person and A/D person to bond. Just be sure to check in often.

If the relief caregiver is new, it is best to have trusted friends or family drop by unannounced on occasion just to see how things are going. It's great if you can find someone with good references from people you know. But not every pairing works and don't hesitate to find someone else if your family member is apprehensive about being left with the relief caregiver even after several visits. Let your 'gut instinct' be your guide in this. Many times when abusive situations are discovered, family members will say they had a 'feeling' something was wrong, but never acted on it for lack of anything concrete.

Of course, the respite person should be introduced slowly and the primary caregiver should be present for the first couple of visits then leave for an hour or so, increasing the caregiver's time off as needed. Sometimes guilt is experienced at leaving the A/D person 'alone', especially if he/she is upset at first. But every caregiver needs a break now and then. You will be of no use if you allow yourself to become ill from exhaustion.

It's also good to have someone whom your A/D person is comfortable with in case of emergency. You must have a written plan in place, somewhere easy for emergency personnel to find that arranges for the care of the A/D person in case the caregiver has an emergency. Give a copy to a trusted person who is the emergency contact person. Too often, caregivers are so caught up in the day to day routine, they don't stop to think about what would happen should THEY be the one to suddenly fall ill.

CAREGIVING

And that leads us to our most important chapter of all: for the caregiver. The twenty-four hours a day, seven days a week, three hundred and sixty-five days a year care giving job is exhausting, period. You must take care of yourself. Killing yourself to take care of others is a bad thing. If you are exhausted you are of little help and may miss important clues in the health of your A/D person because you were too tired to notice.

If you are reading this and letting someone else in the family do most of the day to day care, you must take the time to give them as much help and support as you possibly can. Often family members don't realize the primary caregiver needs help until a crisis occurs. Don't be one of those families. Please.

It is often the case that most of the care falls to one or two people; perhaps they have a more flexible schedule or other family members can not risk taking time off work. If you are one the latter group, then you can contribute financially so the regular caregiver feels he/she can afford to hire a respite person. But everyone in the family that has the means to do so should contribute in some way.

Most states have some sort of Senior Services Division through the Department of Health and Human Services. Often, a social worker will come out to your home, evaluate the situation and give you information on state and federal programs available to help provide in home care for A/D persons.

Some states have more services available than others, but government is realizing that seniors and those with A/D get better care, stay healthier longer and cost less to care for when they are at home. You contacting your state's Senior Services Department and finding out what help is available is one of the most important things that you as a caregiver can do for yourself and your A/D person.

One moral issue caregivers face is how much information to give and when to omit things or change stories. Great guilt is felt when a person feels they are 'lying' to the loved one. But is it kind to tell someone their best friend is dead and watch them go through grief over and over because they don't remember that you told them yesterday?

Difficult issues can be addressed without being dishonest. It is not lying to say, "Let's not go visit Jack today, he isn't home". "Where is he?" "I can't say, but he is not there, that much I do know." Sometimes leaving things out is just kinder.

Diseased brains often struggle to comprehend even simple matters. Only the most basic information is all they can handle. If the person is getting agitated as you give details, please stop. He/she can't properly process them. Keeping it simple is kinder to them and less stressful for you.

LEGAL ISSUES

If Early Onset A/D is involved and it is necessary to file for Social Security Disability, assembling all the medical records and other documentation yourself before hand can save on fees. Make sure you contract with a reputable legal firm that specializes in disability claims, although often legal counsel is not sought until after the initial claim has been rejected. If the Alzheimer's victim is turned down on the first hearing, don't despair. Seek legal help and appeal until you get a favorable decision.

Occasionally, in severe a case of disability, a claim is approved the first go around, but it often takes three or more tries to be approved. It seems to be built into the system to make getting benefits difficult. Unscrupulous people have made this system necessary to help stop fraud.

Having good documentation will help your case. Multiple specialists documenting that your loved one is incapable of working seems to help. Just don't give up. Keep appealing until you get a fair decision. After all, your A/D person has paid into the system to be financially compensated if he/she is unable to work.

Another issue that may require legal advice is the management of financial affairs. Many A/D people have difficulty managing finances and are easy prey for those who would take advantage of the frail. Although talking money issues is difficult in our society, arrangements should be made while your loved one is still competent to sign documents giving Power of Attorney to handle the finances to a trusted person, often the caregiver.

Someone has to be sure the bills get paid, needs are cared for, services obtained through state and local agencies, and insurances billed. The maze of paperwork that comes with long term illness can be mind boggling. Don't hesitate to ask for help from a trusted friend, loved one or legal adviser if needed. Some states can arrange a payee to take care of the financial responsibilities if needed. Your local senior services agency can be helpful in locating a trustworthy payee if circumstances require it.

Many older people have Durable Power of Attorneys arranged with their legal adviser for just such issues. But if you have not, please take care of it right away. It is much more pleasant to do this in a private setting than it is to go to court later to have the loved one ruled incompetent to handle his or her own affairs.

In everything regarding legal issues, seek the advice of an attorney who specializes in these matters.

CONCLUSION

Lastly, take the time to educate yourself. New research comes out on a regular basis. Stay on top of the latest nutrition and keep in touch with your local, state and county services workers, who will often be a valuable resource for information on the latest programs available to you. Keep doing the activities that you love. Enjoy the time you have with your loved one. And remember to laugh now and then.

It is our sincere hope that this is helpful to you in some way. We care deeply about the suffering Alzheimer's victims, their families and loved ones go through trying to cope with this relentless, devastating disease.

Perhaps this book has brought a ray of hope into your life.

Notes

About The Author

For more than thirty-five years, Karen McCormick has been obsessed with nutrition and its role in maximizing the body's ability to heal itself. As an Army medic and then working in teaching hospitals as a nursing assistant, she heard stories of miraculous healing where there was no hope, often aided by intense nutritional focus. Not bound by the belief that it takes a drug to cure an illness, she began to investigate on her own and came to realize there is much we, as the owners of our bodies, can do to be in a healthy state and avoid disease. She believes we must work with our physicians as part of a team and that the patient has just as much responsibility to do their part as the physician does in the healing process.

Since that time, she has continued to explore and learn, sharing her knowledge with family and friends. Now she has branched out to share the word of hope and healing to others in this first publication, Alzheimer's Healing".